I0483786

Guidelines for Nursing Homes
Ergonomics for the Prevention
of Musculoskeletal Disorders

U.S. Department of Labor
Elaine L. Chao, Secretary

Occupational Safety and Health Administration
John L. Henshaw, Assistant Secretary

OSHA 3182-3R 2009

Table of Contents

Table of Contents

Executive Summary

These guidelines provide recommendations for nursing home employers to help reduce the number and severity of work-related musculoskeletal disorders (MSDs) in their facilities. MSDs include conditions such as low back pain, sciatica, rotator cuff injuries, epicondylitis, and carpal tunnel syndrome. The recommendations in these guidelines are based on a review of existing practices and programs, State OSHA programs, as well as available scientific information, and reflect comments received from representatives of trade and professional associations, labor organizations, the medical community, individual firms, and other interested parties. OSHA thanks the many organizations and individuals involved for their thoughtful comments, suggestions, and assistance.

More remains to be learned about the relationship between workplace activities and the development of MSDs. However, OSHA believes that the experiences of many nursing homes provide a basis for taking action to better protect workers. As the understanding of these injuries develops and information and technology improve, the recommendations made in this document may be modified.

Although these guidelines are designed specifically for nursing homes, OSHA hopes that employers with similar work environments, such as assisted living centers, homes for the disabled, homes for the aged, and hospitals will also find this information useful.

OSHA also recognizes that small employers, in particular, may not have the need for as comprehensive a program as would result from implementation of every action and strategy described in these guidelines. Additionally, OSHA realizes that many small employers may need assistance in implementing an appropriate ergonomics program. That is why we emphasize the availability of the free OSHA consultation service for smaller employers. The consultation service is independent of OSHA's enforcement activity and will be making special efforts to provide help to the nursing home industry.

These guidelines are advisory in nature and informational in content. They are not a new standard or regulation and do not create any new OSHA duties. Under the OSH Act, the extent of an employer's obligation to address ergonomic hazards is governed by the general duty clause, 29 U.S.C. 654(a)(1).

An employer's failure to implement the guidelines is not a violation, or evidence of a violation, and may not be used as evidence of a violation, of the general duty clause. Furthermore, the fact that OSHA has developed this document is not evidence and may not be used as evidence of an employer's obligations under the general duty clause; the fact that a measure is recommended in this document but not adopted by an employer is not evidence, and may not be used as evidence, of a violation of the general duty clause. In addition, the recommendations contained herein should be adapted to the needs and resources of each individual place of employment. Thus, implementation of the guidelines may differ from site to site depending on the circumstances at each particular site.

While specific measures may differ from site to site, OSHA recommends that:

- **Manual lifting of residents be minimized in all cases and eliminated when feasible.**
- **Employers implement an effective ergonomics process that:**
  - **provides management support;**
  - **involves employees;**
  - **identifies problems;**
  - **implements solutions;**
  - **addresses reports of injuries;**
  - **provides training; and**
  - **evaluates ergonomics efforts.**

These guidelines elaborate on these recommendations, and include additional information employers can use to identify problems and train employees. Of particular value are examples of solutions employers can use to help reduce MSDs in their workplace. Recommended solutions for resident lifting and repositioning are found in Section III, while recommended solutions for other ergonomic concerns are in Section IV. The appendix includes a case study describing the process one nursing home used to reduce MSDs.

Introduction

Nursing homes that have implemented injury prevention efforts focusing on resident lifting and repositioning methods have achieved considerable success in reducing work-related injuries and associated workers' compensation costs. Providing a safer and more comfortable work environment has also resulted in additional benefits for some facilities, including reduced staff turnover and associated training and administrative costs, reduced absenteeism, increased productivity, improved employee morale, and increased resident comfort. These guidelines provide recommendations for employers to help them reduce the number and severity of work-related musculoskeletal disorders in their facilities using methods that have been found to be successful in the nursing home environment.

Providing care to nursing home residents is physically demanding work. Nursing home residents often require assistance to walk, bathe, or perform other normal daily activities. In some cases residents are totally dependent upon caregivers for mobility. Manual lifting and other tasks involving the repositioning of residents are associated with an increased risk of pain and injury to caregivers, particularly to the back (2, 3). These tasks can entail high physical demands due to the large amount of weight involved, awkward postures that may result from leaning over a bed or working in a confined area, shifting of weight that may occur if a resident loses balance or strength while moving, and many other factors. The risk factors that workers in nursing homes face include:

- Force - the amount of physical effort required to perform a task (such as heavy lifting) or to maintain control of equipment or tools;
- Repetition - performing the same motion or series of motions continually or frequently; and
- Awkward postures - assuming positions that place stress on the body, such as reaching above shoulder height, kneeling, squatting, leaning over a bed, or twisting the torso while lifting (3).

Wyandot County Nursing Home in Upper Sandusky, Ohio, has implemented a policy of performing all assisted resident transfers with mechanical lifts, and has purchased electrically adjustable beds. According to Wyandot, no back injuries from resident lifting have occurred in over five years. The nursing home also reported that workers' compensation costs have declined from an average of almost $140,000 per year to less than $4,000 per year, reduced absenteeism and overtime have resulted in annual savings of approximately $55,000, and a reduction in costs associated with staff turnover has saved an additional $125,000 (1). (see Reference List)

Introduction

Excessive exposure to these risk factors can result in a variety of disorders in affected workers (3, 5). These conditions are collectively referred to as musculoskeletal disorders, or MSDs. MSDs include conditions such as low back pain, sciatica, rotator cuff injuries, epicondylitis, and carpal tunnel syndrome (6). Early indications of MSDs can include persistent pain, restriction of joint movement, or soft tissue swelling (3, 7).

While some MSDs develop gradually over time, others may result from instantaneous events such as a single heavy lift (3). Activities outside of the workplace that involve substantial physical demands may also cause or contribute to MSDs (6). In addition, development of MSDs may be related to genetic causes, gender, age, and other factors (5, 6). Finally, there is evidence that reports of MSDs may be linked to certain psychosocial factors such as job dissatisfaction, monotonous work, and limited job control (5, 6). These guidelines address only physical factors in the workplace that are related to the development of MSDs.

After implementing a program designed to eliminate manual lifting of residents, Schoellkopf Health Center in Niagara Falls, New York, reported a downward trend in the number and severity of injuries, with lost workdays dropping from 364 to 52, light duty days dropping from 253 to 25, and workers' compensation losses falling from $84,533 to $6,983 annually (4).

At Citizens Memorial Health Care Facility in Bolivar, Missouri, establishment of an ergonomics component in the existing safety and health program was reportedly followed by a reduction in the number of OSHA-recordable lifting-related injuries of at least 45% during each of the next four years, when compared to the level of injuries prior to the ergonomics efforts. The number of lost workdays associated with lifting-related injuries was reported to be at least 55% lower than levels during each of the previous four years. Citizens Memorial reported that these reductions contributed to a direct savings of approximately $150,000 in workers' compensation costs over a five year period (8).

SECTION II
A Process for Protecting Workers

The number and severity of injuries resulting from physical demands in nursing homes — and associated costs — can be substantially reduced (2, 9). Providing an alternative to manual resident lifting is the primary goal of the ergonomics process in the nursing home setting and of these guidelines. **OSHA recommends that manual lifting of residents be minimized in all cases and eliminated when feasible.** OSHA further recommends that employers develop a process for systematically addressing ergonomics issues in their facilities, and incorporate this process into an overall program to recognize and prevent occupational safety and health hazards.

An effective process should be tailored to the characteristics of the particular nursing home but OSHA generally recommends the following steps:

Provide Management Support

Strong support by management creates the best opportunity for success. OSHA recommends that employers develop clear goals, assign responsibilities to designated staff members to achieve those goals, provide necessary resources, and ensure that assigned responsibilities are fulfilled. Providing a safe and healthful workplace requires a sustained effort, allocation of resources, and frequent follow-up that can only be achieved through the active support of management.

Involve Employees

Employees are a vital source of information about hazards in their workplace. Their involvement adds problem-solving capabilities and hazard identification assistance, enhances worker motivation and job satisfaction, and leads to greater acceptance when changes are made in the workplace. Employees can:

- submit suggestions or concerns;
- discuss the workplace and work methods;
- participate in the design of work, equipment, procedures, and training;
- evaluate equipment;
- respond to employee surveys;
- participate in task groups with responsibility for ergonomics; and
- participate in developing the nursing home's ergonomics process.

A Process for Protecting Workers

An Identify Problems

Nursing homes can more successfully recognize problems by establishing systematic methods for identifying ergonomics concerns in their workplace. Information about where problems or potential problems may occur in nursing homes can be obtained from a variety of sources, including OSHA 300 and 301 injury and illness information, reports of workers' compensation claims, accident and near-miss investigation reports, insurance company reports, employee interviews, employee surveys, and reviews and observations of workplace conditions. Once information is obtained, it can be used to identify and evaluate elements of jobs that are associated with problems. Sections III and IV contain further information on methods for identifying ergonomics concerns in the nursing home environment.

Implement Solutions

When problems related to ergonomics are identified, suitable options can then be selected and implemented to eliminate hazards. Effective solutions usually involve workplace modifications that eliminate hazards and improve the work environment. These changes usually include the use of equipment, work practices, or both. When choosing methods for lifting and repositioning residents, individual factors should be taken into account. Such factors include the resident's rehabilitation plan, the need to restore the resident's functional abilities, medical contraindications, emergency situations, and resident dignity and rights. Examples of solutions can be found in Sections III and IV.

Address Reports of Injuries

Even in establishments with effective safety and health programs, injuries and illnesses may occur. Work-related MSDs should be managed in the same manner and under the same process as any other occupational injury or illness (10). Like many injuries and illnesses, employers and employees can benefit from early reporting of MSDs. Early diagnosis and intervention, including alternative duty programs, are particularly important in order to limit the severity of injury, improve the effectiveness of treatment, minimize the likelihood of disability or permanent damage, and reduce the amount of associated workers' compensation claims and costs. OSHA's injury and illness recording and reporting regulation (29 CFR 1904) requires employers to keep records of work-related injuries and illnesses. These reports can help the nursing home identify problem areas and evaluate ergonomic efforts. Employees may not be discriminated against for reporting a work-related injury or illness. [29 U.S.C. 660(c)]

Provide Training

Training is necessary to ensure that employees and managers can recognize potential ergonomics issues in the workplace, and understand measures that are available to minimize the risk of injury. Ergonomics training can be integrated into general training on performance requirements and job practices. Effective training covers the problems found in each employee's job. More information on training can be found in Section V.

Evaluate Ergonomics Efforts

Nursing homes should evaluate the effectiveness of their ergonomics efforts and follow-up on unresolved problems. Evaluation helps sustain the effort to reduce injuries and illnesses, track whether or not ergonomic solutions are working, identify new problems, and show areas where further improvement is needed. Evaluation and follow-up are central to continuous improvement and long-term success. Once solutions are introduced, OSHA recommends that employers ensure they are effective. Various indicators (e.g., OSHA 300 and 301 information data and workers' compensation reports) can provide useful empirical data at this stage, as can other techniques such as employee interviews. For example, after introducing a new lift at a nursing home, the employer should follow-up by talking with employees to ensure that the problem has been adequately addressed. In addition, interviews provide a mechanism for ensuring that the solution is not only in place, but is being used properly. The same methods that are used to identify problems in many cases can also be used for evaluation.

A Identifying Problems and Implementing Solutions for Resident Lifting and Repositioning

Identifying Problems for Resident Lifting and Repositioning

Assessing the potential for work to injure employees in nursing homes is complex because typical nursing home operations involve the repeated lifting and repositioning of the residents. Resident lifting and repositioning tasks can be variable, dynamic, and unpredictable in nature. In addition, factors such as resident dignity, safety, and medical contraindications should be taken into account. As a result, specific techniques are used for assessing resident lifting and repositioning tasks that are not appropriate for assessing the potential for injury associated with other nursing home activities.

An analysis of any resident lifting and repositioning task involves an assessment of the needs and abilities of the resident involved. This assessment allows staff members to account for resident characteristics while determining the safest methods for performing the task, within the context of a care plan that provides for appropriate care and services for the resident. Such assessments typically consider the resident's safety, dignity and other rights, as well as the need to maintain or restore a resident's functional abilities.

The resident assessment should include examination of factors such as:

- the level of assistance the resident requires;
- the size and weight of the resident;
- the ability and willingness of the resident to understand and cooperate; and
- any medical conditions that may influence the choice of methods for lifting or repositioning.

These factors are critically important in determining appropriate methods for lifting and repositioning a resident. The size and weight of the resident will, in some situations, determine which equipment is needed and how many caregivers are required to provide assistance. The physical and mental abilities of the resident also play an important role in selecting appropriate solutions. For example, a resident who is able and willing to partially support their own weight may be able to move from his or her bed to a chair using a standing assist device, while a mechanical sling lift may be more appropriate for those residents who are unable to support their own weight. Other factors related to a resident's condition may need to be taken into account as well. For instance, a resident who has recently undergone hip replacement surgery may require specialized equipment for assistance in order to avoid placing stress on the affected area.

A number of protocols have been developed for systematically examining resident needs and abilities and/or

Identifying Problems and Implementing Solutions
for Resident Lifting and Repositioning

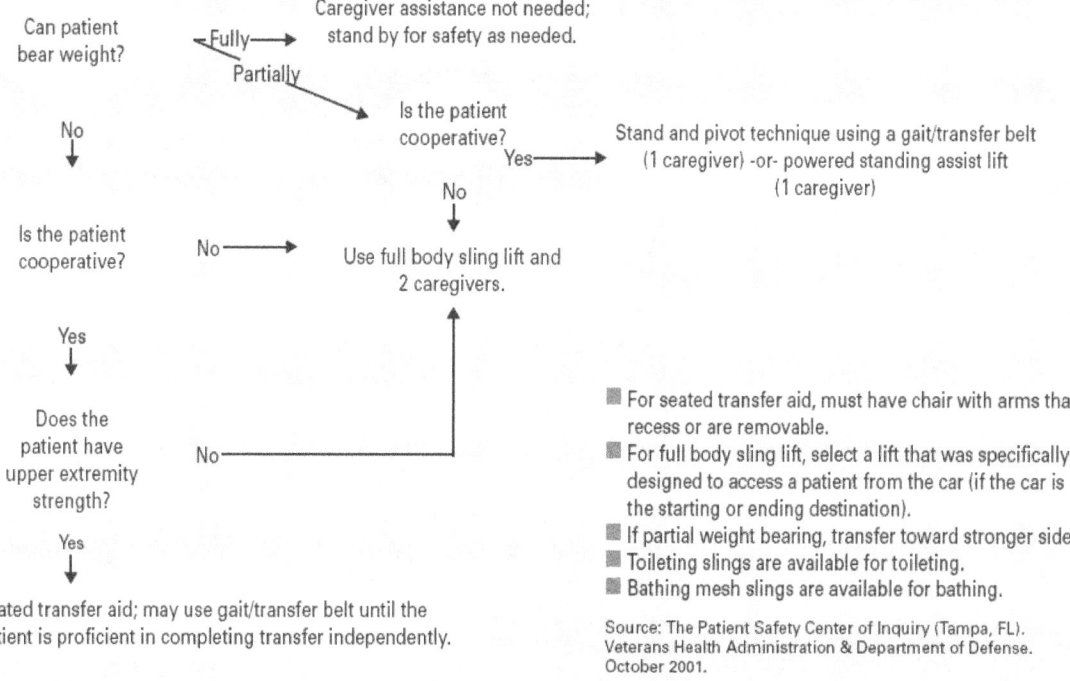

For seated transfer aid, must have chair with arms that recess or are removable.

For full body sling lift, select a lift that was specifically designed to access a patient from the car (if the car is the starting or ending destination).

If partial weight bearing, transfer toward stronger side.

Toileting slings are available for toileting.

Bathing mesh slings are available for bathing.

Source: The Patient Safety Center of Inquiry (Tampa, FL). Veterans Health Administration & Department of Defense. October 2001.

FIGURE 2 Lateral Transfer to and from: Bed to Stretcher, Trolley

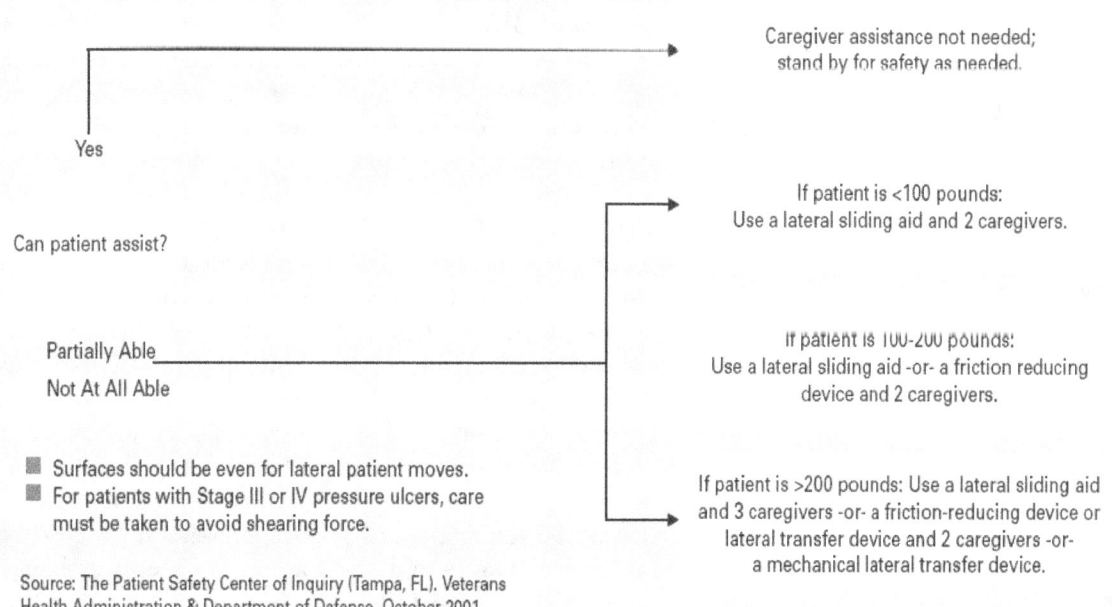

Surfaces should be even for lateral patient moves.

For patients with Stage III or IV pressure ulcers, care must be taken to avoid shearing force.

Source: The Patient Safety Center of Inquiry (Tampa, FL). Veterans Health Administration & Department of Defense. October 2001.

Identifying Problems and Implementing Solutions for Resident Lifting and Repositioning

for recommending procedures and equipment to be used for performing lifting and repositioning tasks. The following are some examples:

- The *Resident Assessment Instrument*, published by the Centers for Medicare and Medicaid Services (CMS), provides a structured, standardized approach for assessing resident capabilities and needs that results in a care plan for each resident. Caregivers can use this information to help them determine the appropriate method for lifting or repositioning residents. Many nursing homes use this system to comply with CMS requirements for nursing homes. Employers can access this information from www.cms.hhs.gov/medicaid/mds20/.

- *Patient Care Ergonomics Resource Guide: Safe Patient Handling and Movement* is published by the Patient Safety Center of Inquiry, Veterans Health Administration and the Department of Defense. This document provides flow charts (shown here in Figures 1-6) that address relevant resident assessment factors and recommends solutions for resident lifting and repositioning problems. This material is one example of an assessment tool that has been used successfully. Employers can access this information from www.patientsafetycenter.com. Nursing home operators may find another tool or develop an assessment tool that works better in their facilities.

- Appendix A of the Settlement Agreement between OSHA and Beverly Enterprises, entitled *Lift*

Program Policy and Guide, recommends solutions for resident lifting and repositioning problems, based on the CMS classification system. (A rating of "4" indicates a totally dependent resident; a "3" rating indicates residents that need extensive assistance; a "2/1" rating indicates residents that need only limited assistance/general supervision. Residents rated "0" are independent.) Employers can access this information from www.osha.gov.

The nursing home operator should use an assessment tool which is appropriate for the conditions in an individual nursing home. The special needs of bariatric (excessively heavy) residents may require additional focus. Assistive devices must be capable of handling the heavier weight involved, and modification of work practices may be necessary. A number of individuals in nursing homes can contribute to resident assessment and the determination of appropriate methods for assisting in transfer or repositioning. Interdisciplinary teams such as staff nurses, certified nursing assistants, nursing supervisors, physical therapists, physicians, and the resident or his/her representative may all be involved. Of critical importance is the involvement of employees directly responsible for resident care and assistance, as the needs and abilities of residents may vary considerably over a short period of time, and the employees responsible for providing assistance are in the best position to be aware of and accommodate such changes.

Identifying Problems and Implementing Solutions
for Resident Lifting and Repositioning

FIGURE 3 Transfer to and from: Chair to Stretcher

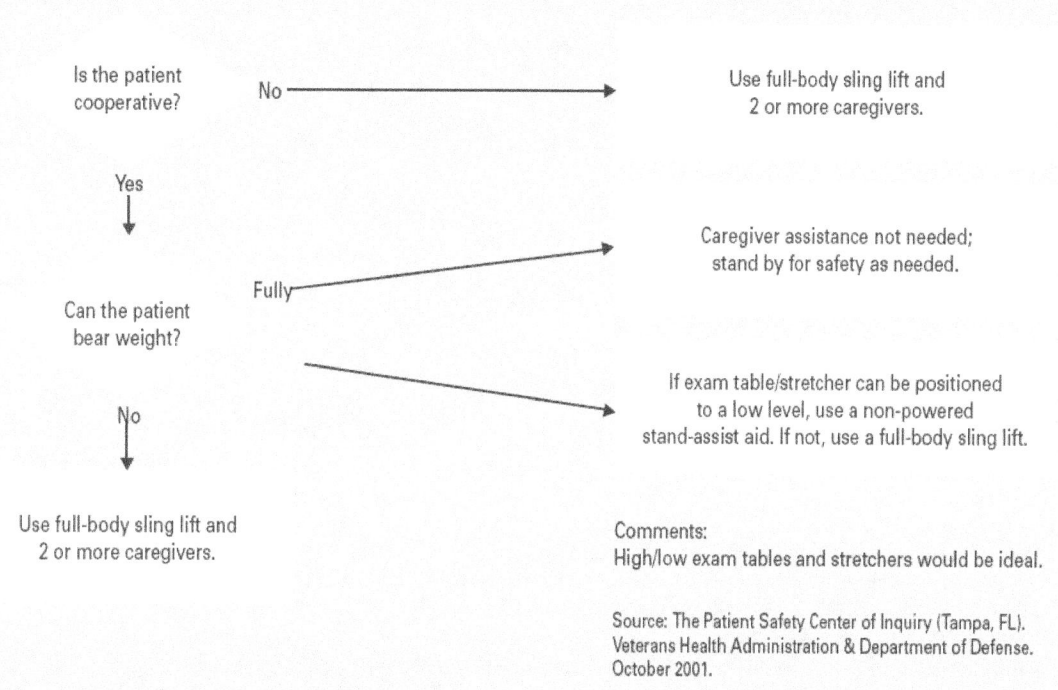

Is the patient cooperative? — No → Use full-body sling lift and 2 or more caregivers.

Yes ↓

Can the patient bear weight? — Fully → Caregiver assistance not needed; stand by for safety as needed.

If exam table/stretcher can be positioned to a low level, use a non-powered stand-assist aid. If not, use a full-body sling lift.

No ↓

Use full-body sling lift and 2 or more caregivers.

Comments:
High/low exam tables and stretchers would be ideal.

Source: The Patient Safety Center of Inquiry (Tampa, FL).
Veterans Health Administration & Department of Defense.
October 2001.

FIGURE 4 Reposition in Bed: Side-to-Side, Up in Bed

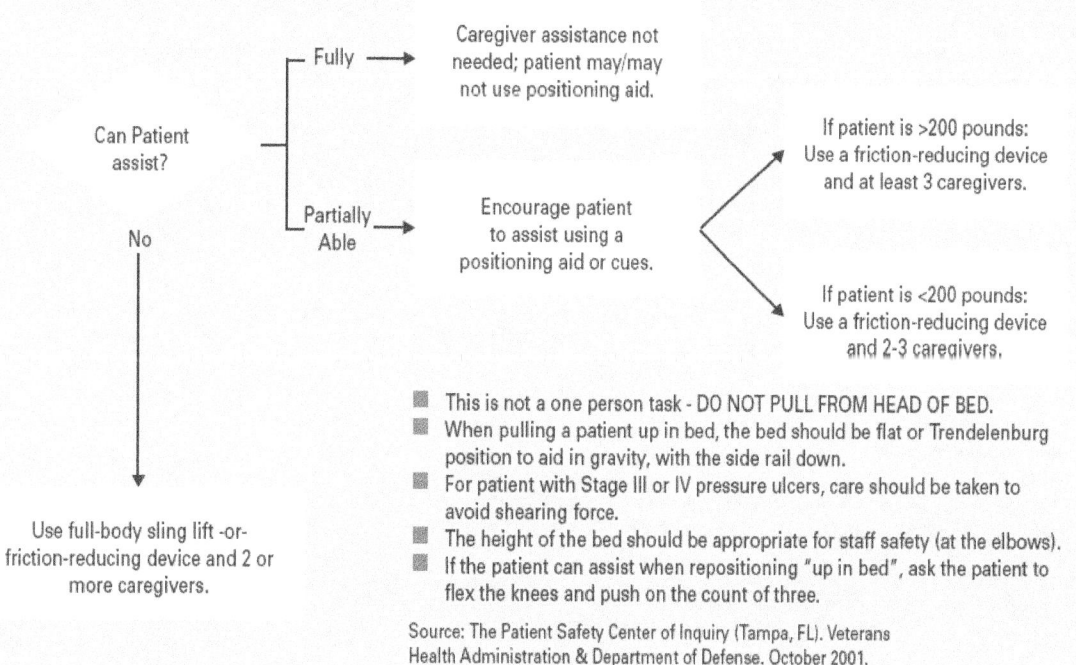

Can Patient assist? — Fully → Caregiver assistance not needed; patient may/may not use positioning aid.

Partially Able → Encourage patient to assist using a positioning aid or cues.

If patient is >200 pounds: Use a friction-reducing device and at least 3 caregivers.

If patient is <200 pounds: Use a friction-reducing device and 2-3 caregivers.

No ↓

Use full-body sling lift -or- friction-reducing device and 2 or more caregivers.

- This is not a one person task - DO NOT PULL FROM HEAD OF BED.
- When pulling a patient up in bed, the bed should be flat or Trendelenburg position to aid in gravity, with the side rail down.
- For patient with Stage III or IV pressure ulcers, care should be taken to avoid shearing force.
- The height of the bed should be appropriate for staff safety (at the elbows).
- If the patient can assist when repositioning "up in bed", ask the patient to flex the knees and push on the count of three.

Source: The Patient Safety Center of Inquiry (Tampa, FL). Veterans
Health Administration & Department of Defense. October 2001.

Identifying Problems and Implementing Solutions
for Resident Lifting and Repositioning

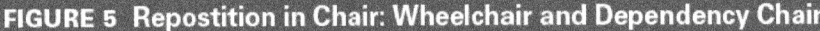

FIGURE 5 Repostition in Chair: Wheelchair and Dependency Chair

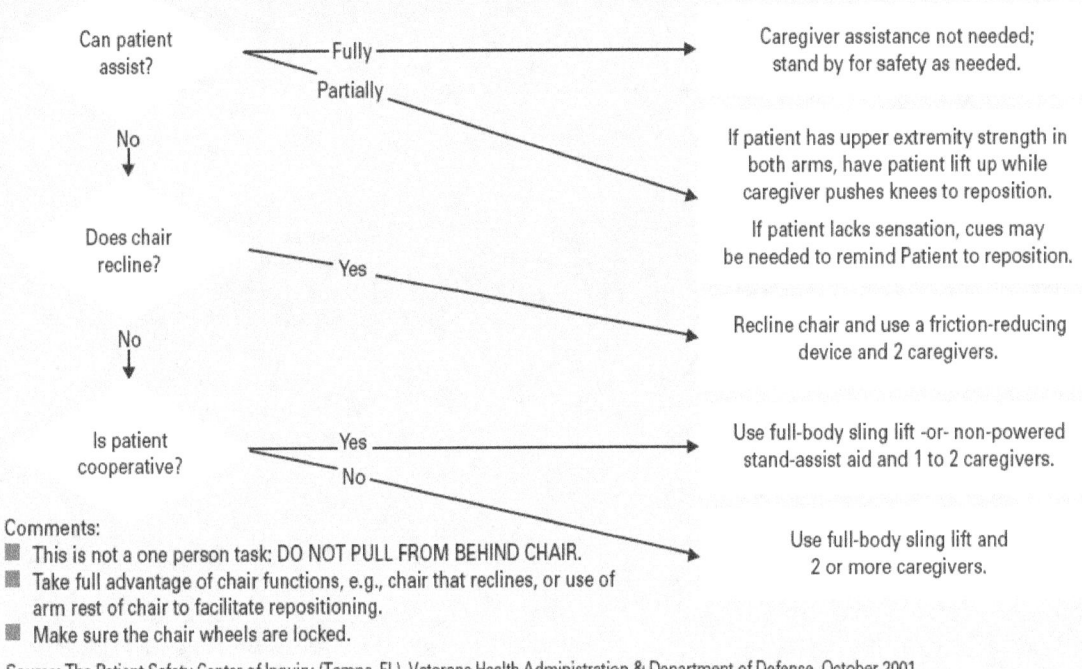

Can patient assist? — Fully → Caregiver assistance not needed; stand by for safety as needed.

Partially → If patient has upper extremity strength in both arms, have patient lift up while caregiver pushes knees to reposition.

If patient lacks sensation, cues may be needed to remind Patient to reposition.

No ↓

Does chair recline? — Yes → Recline chair and use a friction-reducing device and 2 caregivers.

No ↓

Is patient cooperative? — Yes → Use full-body sling lift -or- non-powered stand-assist aid and 1 to 2 caregivers.

No → Use full-body sling lift and 2 or more caregivers.

Comments:
- This is not a one person task: DO NOT PULL FROM BEHIND CHAIR.
- Take full advantage of chair functions, e.g., chair that reclines, or use of arm rest of chair to facilitate repositioning.
- Make sure the chair wheels are locked.

Source: The Patient Safety Center of Inquiry (Tampa, FL). Veterans Health Administration & Department of Defense. October 2001.

FIGURE 6 Transfer a Patient Up From the Floor

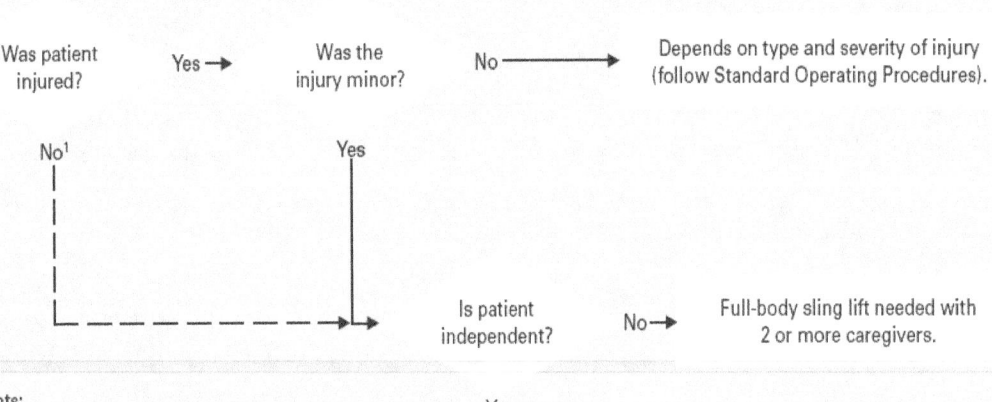

Was patient injured? — Yes → Was the injury minor? — No → Depends on type and severity of injury (follow Standard Operating Procedures).

No[1]

Yes

Is patient independent? — No → Full-body sling lift needed with 2 or more caregivers.

Yes ↓ Caregiver assistance not needed; stand by for safety as needed.

Comments:
Use full-body sling that goes all the way down to the floor (most of the newer models are capable of this).

[1]Modifications made with concurrence of Dr. Audrey Nelson at Veterans Administration Hospital, Tampa, Florida.

Source: The Patient Safety Center of Inquiry (Tampa, FL).
Veterans Health Administration & Department of Defense. October 2001.

Identifying Problems and Implementing Solutions
for Resident Lifting and Repositioning

Implementing Solutions for Resident Lifting and Repositioning

The recommended solutions presented in the following pages are not intended to be an exhaustive list, nor does OSHA expect that all of them will be used in any given facility. The information represents a range of available options that a facility can consider using. Many of the solutions are simple, common sense modifications to equipment or procedures that do not require substantial time or resources to implement. Others may require more significant efforts. The integration of various solutions into the nursing home is a strategic decision that, if carefully planned and executed, will lead to long-term benefits. Equipment must meet applicable regulations regarding equipment design and use, such as the restraint regulations from the Centers for Medicare and Medicaid. In addition, administrators should follow any manufacturers' recommendations and review guidelines, such as the *FDA Hospital Bed Safety Workgroup Guidelines*, to help ensure patient safety. Management should also be cognizant of several factors that might restrict the application of certain measures, such as residents' rehabilitation plans, the need for restoration of functional abilities, other medical contraindications, emergency conditions, and residents' dignity and rights.

The procurement of equipment and the selection of an equipment supplier are important considerations when implementing solutions.

Employers should establish close working relationships with equipment suppliers. Such working relationships help with obtaining training for employees, modifying the equipment for special circumstances, and procuring parts and service when needed. Employers will want to pay particular attention to the effectiveness of the equipment, especially the injury and illness experience of other nursing homes that have used the equipment. The following questions are designed to aid in the selection of the equipment and supplier that best meets the needs of an individual nursing home.

- Availability of technical service - Is over-the-phone assistance, as well as onsite assistance, for repairs and service of the lift available?
- Availability of parts - Which parts will be in stock and available in a short time frame and how soon can they be shipped to your location?
- Storage requirements - Is the equipment too big for your facility? Can it be stored in close proximity to the area(s) where it is used?
- If needed, is a charging unit and back up battery included? What is the simplicity of the charging unit and space required for a battery charger if one is needed?

Identifying Problems and Implementing Solutions for Resident Lifting and Repositioning

- If the lift has a self-contained charging unit, what is the amount of space necessary for charging and what electrical receptacles are required? What is the minimum charging time of a battery?
- How high is the base of the lift and will it fit under the bed and various other pieces of furniture? How wide is the base of the lift or is it adjustable to a wider and lockable position?
- How many people are required to operate the lift for lifting of a typical 200-pound person?
- Does the lift activation device (pendant) have remote capabilities?
- How many sizes and types of slings are available? What type of sling is available for optimum infection control?
- Is the device versatile? Can it be a sit-to-stand lift, as well as a lift device? Can it be a sit-to-stand lift and an ambulation-assist device?
- What is the speed and noise level of the device? Will the lift go to floor level? How high will it go?

Based on many factors, including the characteristics of the resident population and the layout of the facility, employers should determine the number and types of devices needed. Devices should be located so that they are easily accessible to workers. If resident lifting equipment is not accessible when it is needed, it is likely that other aspects of the ergonomics process will be ineffective. If the facility can initially purchase only a portion of the equipment needed, it should be located in the areas where the needs are greatest. Employers should also establish routine maintenance schedules to ensure that the equipment is in good working order.

The following are examples of solutions for resident lifting and repositioning tasks.

Identifying Problems and Implementing Solutions
for Resident Lifting and Repositioning

Transfer from Sitting to Standing Position

Description:
Powered sit-to-stand or standing assist devices.

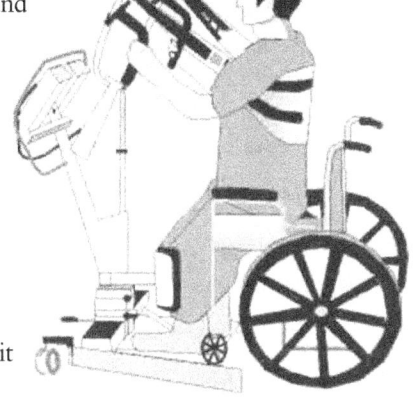

When to Use:
Transferring residents who are partially dependent, have some weight-bearing capacity, are cooperative, can sit up on the edge of the bed with or without assistance, and are able to bend hips, knees, and ankles. Transfers from bed to chair (wheel chair, Geri or cardiac chair), or chair to bed, or for bathing and toileting. Can be used for repositioning where space or storage is limited.

Points to Remember:
Look for a device that has a variety of sling sizes, lift-height range, battery portability, hand-held control, emergency shut-off, and manual override. Ensure device is rated for the resident weight. Electric/battery powered lifts are preferred to crank or pump type devices to allow smoother movement for the resident, and less physical exertion by the caregiver.

Resident Lifting

Description:
Portable lift device (sling type); can be a universal/ hammock sling or a band/ leg sling.

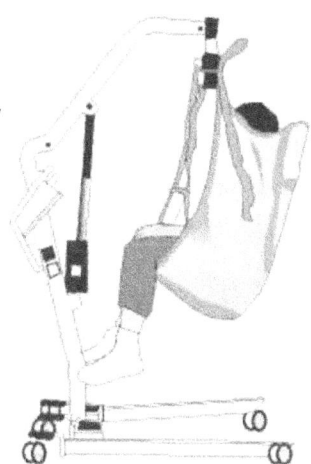

When to Use:
Lifting residents who are totally dependent, are partial- or non-weight bearing, are very heavy, or have other physical limitations. Transfers from bed to chair (wheel chair, Geri or cardiac chair), chair or floor to bed, for bathing and toileting, or after a resident fall.

Points to Remember:
More than one caregiver may be needed. Look for a device with a variety of slings, lift-height range, battery portability, hand-held control, emergency shut-off, manual override, boom pressure sensitive switch, that can easily move around equipment, and has a support base that goes under beds. Having multiple slings allows one of them to remain in place while resident is in bed or chair for only a short period, reducing the number of times the caregiver lifts and positions resident. Portable compact lifts may be useful where space or storage is limited. Ensure device is rated for the resident weight. Electric/battery powered lifts are preferred to crank or pump type devices to allow a smoother movement for the resident, and less physical exertion by the caregiver. Enhances resident safety and comfort.

Repositioning in Chair

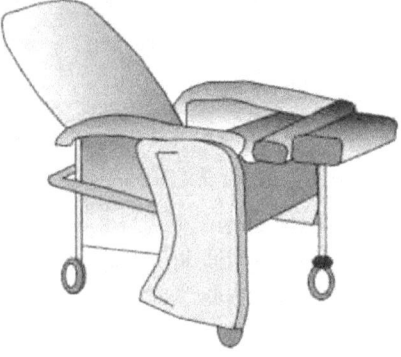

Description:
Variable position Geri and Cardiac chairs.

When to Use:
Repositioning partial- or non-weight-bearing residents who are cooperative.

Points to Remember:
More than one caregiver is needed and use of a friction-reducing device is needed if resident cannot assist to reposition self in chair. Ensure use of good body mechanics by caregivers. Wheels on chair add versatility. Ensure that chair is easy to adjust, move, and steer. Lock wheels on chair before repositioning. Remove trays, footrests, and seat belts where appropriate. Ensure device is rated for the resident weight.

Ambulation

Description:
Ambulation assist device.

When to Use:
For residents who are weight bearing and cooperative and who need extra security and assistance when ambulating.

Points to Remember:
Increases resident safety during ambulation and reduces risk of falls. The device supports residents as they walk and push it along during ambulation. Ensure height adjustment is correct for resident before ambulation. Ensure device is in good working order before use and rated for the resident weight to be lifted. Apply brakes before positioning resident in or releasing resident from device.

Resident Lifting

Description:
Ceiling mounted lift device.

When to Use:
Lifting residents who are totally dependent, are partial- or non-weight bearing, very heavy, or have other physical limitations. Transfers from bed to chair (wheel chair, Geri or cardiac chair), chair or floor to bed, for bathing and toileting, or after a resident falls. A horizontal frame system or litter attached to the ceiling-mounted device can be used when transferring residents who cannot be transferred safely between 2 horizontal surfaces, such as a bed to a stretcher or gurney while lying on their back, using other devices.

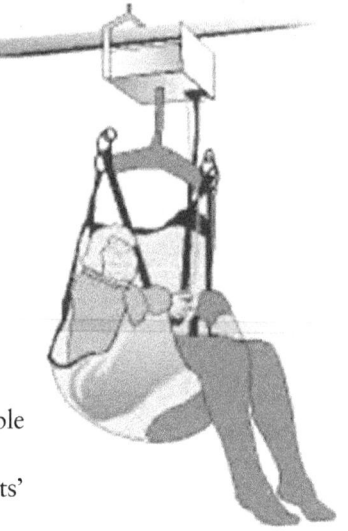

Points to Remember:
More than one caregiver may be needed. Some residents can use the device without assistance. May be quicker to use than portable device. Motors can be fixed or portable (lightweight). Device can be operated by hand-held control attached to unit or by infrared remote control. Ensure device is rated for the resident weight. Increases residents' safety and comfort during transfer.

Lateral Transfer; Repositioning

Description:
Devices to reduce friction force when transferring a resident such as a draw sheet or transfer cot with handles to be used in combination slippery sheets, low friction mattress covers, or slide boards; boards or mats with vinyl coverings and rollers; gurneys with transfer devices; and air-assist lateral sliding aid or flexible mattress inflated by portable air supply.

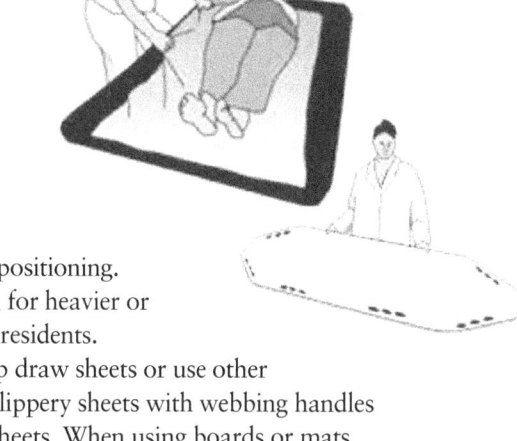

When to Use:
Transferring a partial- or non-weight bearing resident between 2 horizontal surfaces such as a bed to a stretcher or gurney while lying on their back or when repositioning resident in bed.

Points to Remember:
• More than one caregiver is needed to perform this type of transfer or repositioning. Additional assistance may be needed depending upon resident status, e.g., for heavier or non-cooperative residents. Some devices may not be suitable for bariatric residents. When using a draw sheet combination use a good hand-hold by rolling up draw sheets or use other friction-reducing devices with handles such as slippery sheets. Narrower slippery sheets with webbing handles positioned on the long edge of the sheet may be easier to use than wider sheets. When using boards or mats with vinyl coverings and rollers use a gentle push and pull motion to move resident to new surface.
• Look for a combination of devices that will increase resident's comfort and minimize risk of skin trauma. Ensure transfer surfaces are at same level and at a height that allows caregivers to work at waist level to avoid extended reaches and bending of the back. Count down and synchronize the transfer motion between caregivers.

Lateral Transfer; Repositioning

Description:
Convertible wheelchair, Geri or cardiac chair to bed; beds that convert to chairs.

When to Use:
For lateral transfer of residents who are partial- or non-weight bearing. Eliminates the need to perform lift transfer in and out of wheelchairs. Can also be used to assist residents who are partially weight bearing from a sit-to-stand position. Beds that convert to chairs can aid repositioning residents who are totally dependent, non-weight bearing, very heavy, or have other physical limitations.

Points to Remember:
More than one caregiver is needed to perform lateral transfer. Additional assistance for lateral transfer may be needed depending on residents status, e.g., for heavier or non-cooperative residents. Additional friction-reducing devices may be required to reposition resident. Heavy duty beds are available for bariatric residents. Device should have easy-to-use controls located within easy reach of the caregiver, sufficient foot clearance, and wide range of adjustment. Motorized height adjustable devices are preferred to those adjusted by crank mechanism to minimize physical exertion. Always ensure device is in good working order before use. Ensure wheels on equipment are locked. Ensure transfer surfaces are at same level and at a height that allows caregivers to work at waist level to avoid extended reaches and bending of the back.

Lateral Transfer in Sitting Position

Description:
Transfer boards – wood or plastic (some with movable seat).

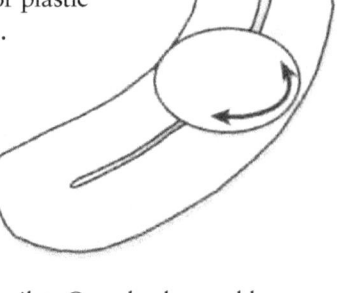

When to Use:
Transferring (sliding) residents who have good sitting balance and are cooperative from one level surface to another, e.g., bed to wheelchair, wheelchair to car seat or toilet. Can also be used by residents who require limited assistance but need additional safety and support.

Points to Remember:
Movable seats increase resident comfort and reduce incidence of tissue damage during transfer. More than one caregiver is needed to perform lateral transfer. Ensure clothing is present between the resident's skin and the transfer device. The seat may be cushioned with a small towel for comfort. May be uncomfortable for larger residents. Usually used in conjunction with gait belts for safety depending on resident status. Ensure boards have tapered ends, rounded edges, and appropriate weight capacity. Ensure wheels on bed or chair are locked and transfer surfaces are at same level. Remove lower bedrails from bed and remove arms and footrests from chairs as appropriate.

Transfer from Sitting to Standing Position

Description:
Stand-assist devices can be fixed to bed or chair or be free-standing. There is a variety of such devices on the market.

When to Use:
Transferring residents who are weight-bearing and cooperative and can pull themselves up from sitting to standing position. Can be used for independent residents who need extra support to stand.

Points to Remember:
Check that device is stable before use and is rated for resident weight to be supported. Ensure frame is firmly attached to bed, or if it relies on mattress support that mattress is heavy enough to hold the frame. Can aid resident independence.

Transfer from Sitting to Standing Position

Description:
Lift cushions and lift chairs.

When to Use:
Transferring residents who are weight-bearing and cooperative but need assistance when standing and ambulating. Can be used for independent residents who need an extra boost to stand.

Points to Remember:
Lift cushions use a lever that activates a spring action to assist residents to rise up. Lift cushions may not be appropriate for heavier residents. Lift chairs are operated via a hand-held control that tilts forward slowly, raising the resident. Residents need to have physical and cognitive capacity to be able to operate lever or controls. Always ensure device is in good working order before use and is rated for the resident weight to be lifted. Can aid resident independence.

Weighing

Description:
Scales with ramp to accommodate wheelchairs; portable-powered lift devices with built-in scales; beds with built-in scales.

When to Use:
To reduce the need for additional transfer of partialor non-weight-bearing or totally dependent residents to weighing device.

Points to Remember:
Some wheelchair scales can accommodate larger wheelchairs. Built-in bed scales may increase weight of the bed and prevent it from lowering to appropriate work heights.

Transfer from Sitting to Standing Position; Ambulation

Description:
Gait belts/transfer belts with handles.

When to Use:
Transferring residents who are partially dependent, have some weight-bearing capacity, and are cooperative. Transfers such as bed to chair, chair to chair, or chair to car; when repositioning residents in chairs; supporting residents during ambulation; and in some cases when guiding and controlling falls or assisting a resident after a fall.

Points to Remember:
• More than one caregiver may be needed. Belts with padded handles are easier to grip and increase security and control. Always transfer to resident's strongest side. Use good body mechanics and a rocking and pulling motion rather than lifting when using a belt. Belts may not be suitable for ambulation of heavy residents or residents with recent abdominal or back surgery, abdominal aneurysm, etc. Should not be used for lifting residents. Ensure belt is securely fastened and cannot be easily undone by the resident during transfer. Ensure a layer of clothing is between residents' skin and the belt to avoid abrasion. Keep resident as close as possible to caregiver during transfer. Lower bedrails, remove arms and foot rests from chairs, and other items that may obstruct the transfer.
• For use after a fall, always assess the resident for injury prior to movement. If resident can regain standing position with minimal assistance, use gait or transfer belts with handles to aid resident. Keep back straight, bend legs, and stay as close to resident as possible.
If resident cannot stand with minimal assistance, use a powered portable or ceiling-mounted lift device to move resident.

Repositioning

Description:
Electric powered height adjustable bed.

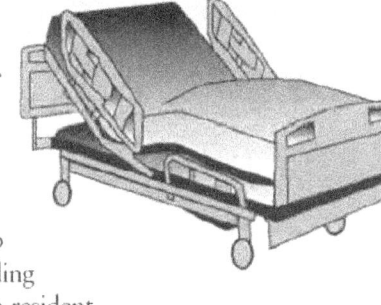

When to Use:
For all activities involving resident care, transfer, repositioning in bed, etc., to reduce caregiver bending when interacting with resident.

Points to Remember:
Device should have easy-to-use controls located within easy reach of the caregiver to promote use of the electric adjustment, sufficient foot clearance, and wide range of adjustment. Adjustments must be completed in 20 seconds or less to ensure staff use. For residents that may be at risk of falling from bed some beds that lower closer to the floor may be needed. Heavy duty beds are available for bariatric residents. Beds raised and lowered with an electric motor are preferred over crank-adjust beds to allow a smoother movement for the resident and less physical exertion to the caregiver.

Repositioning

Description:
Trapeze bar; hand blocks and push up bars attached to the bed frame.

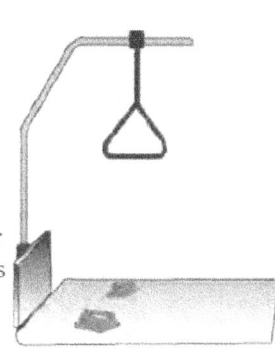

When to Use:
Reposition residents that have the ability to assist the caregiver during the activity, i.e., residents with upper body strength and use of extremities, who are cooperative and can follow instructions.

Points to Remember:
Residents use trapeze bar by grasping bar suspended from an overhead frame to raise themselves up and reposition themselves in a bed. Heavy duty trapeze frames are available for bariatric residents. If a caregiver is assisting, ensure that bed wheels are locked, bedrails are lowered, and bed is adjusted to caregiver's waist height. Blocks also enable residents to raise themselves up and reposition themselves in bed. Bars attached to the bed frame serve the same purpose. May not be suitable for heavier residents. Can aid resident independence.

Repositioning

Description:
Pelvic lift devices (hip lifters).

When to Use:
To assist residents who are cooperative and can sit up to a position on a special bed pan.

Points to Remember:
Convenience of device may reduce need for resident lifting during toileting. Device is positioned under the pelvis. The part of the device located under the pelvis gets inflated so the pelvis is raised and a special bedpan put underneath. The head of the bed is raised slightly during this procedure. Use correct body mechanics, lower bedrails, and adjust bed to caregivers waist height to reduce bending.

Bathtub, Shower, and Toileting Activities

Description:
Height adjustable bathtub and easy-entry bathtubs.

When to Use:
Bathing residents who sit directly in the bathtub, or to assist ambulatory residents climb more easily into a low tub, or easy-access tub. Bathing residents in portable-powered or ceiling mounted lift device using appropriate bathing sling.

Points to Remember:
Reduces awkward postures for caregivers and those who clean the tub after use. The tub can be raised to eliminate bending and reaching for the caregiver. Use correct body mechanics, and adjust the tub to the caregiver's waist height when performing hygiene activities. Increases resident safety and comfort.

Bathtub, Shower, and Toileting Activities

Description:
Shower and toileting chairs.

When to Use:
Showering and toileting residents who are partially dependent, have some weight bearing capacity, can sit up unaided, and are able to bend hips, knees, and ankles.

Points to Remember:
Ensure that wheels move easily and smoothly; chair is high enough to fit over toilet; chair has removable arms, adjustable footrests, safety belts, and is heavy enough to be stable; and that the seat is comfortable, accommodates larger residents, and has a removable commode bucket for toileting. Ensure that brakes lock and hold effectively and that weight capacity is sufficient.

Bathtub, Shower, and Toileting Activities

Description:
Toilet seat risers.

When to Use:
For toileting partially weight-bearing residents who can sit up unaided, use upper extremities (have upper body strength), are able to bend hips, knees, and ankles, and are cooperative. Independent residents can also use these devices.

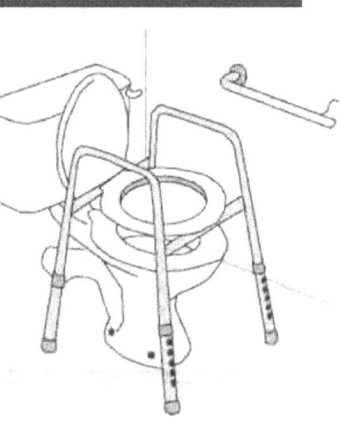

Points to Remember:
Risers decrease the distance and amount of effort required to lower and raise residents. Grab bars and height-adjustable legs add safety and versatility to the device. Ensure device is stable and can accommodate resident's weight and size.

Bathtub, Shower, and Toileting Activities

Description:
Bath boards and transfer benches.

When to Use:
Bathing residents who are partially weight bearing, have good sitting balance, can use upper extremities (have upper body strength), are cooperative, and can follow instructions. Independent residents can also use these devices.

Points to Remember:
To reduce friction and possible skin tears, use clothing or material between the resident's skin and the board. Can be used with a gait or transfer belt and/or grab bars to aid transfer. Back support and vinyl padded seats add to bathing comfort. Look for devices that allow for water drainage and have height-adjustable legs. May not be suitable for heavy residents. If wheelchair is used, ensure wheels are locked, the transfer surfaces are at the same level, and device is securely in place and rated for weight to be transferred. Remove arms and foot rests from chairs as appropriate and ensure that floor is dry.

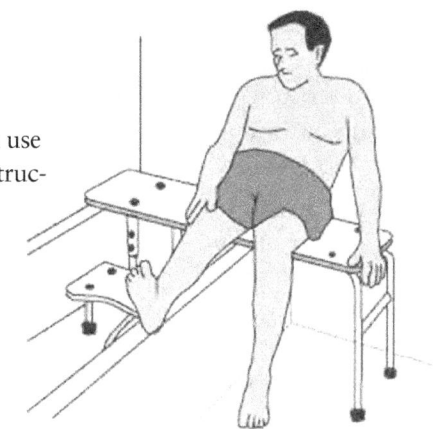

Bathtub, Shower, and Toileting Activities

Description:
Grab bars and stand assists; can be fixed or mobile.

Long-handled or extended shower heads, or brushes can be used for personal hygiene.

When to Use:
Bars and assists help when toileting, bathing, and/ or showering residents who need extra support and security. Residents must be partially weight bearing, able to use upper extremities (have upper body strength), and be cooperative.

Long-handled devices reduce the amount of bending, reaching, and twisting required by the caregiver when washing feet, legs, and trunk of residents. Independent residents who have difficulty reaching lower extremities can also use these devices.

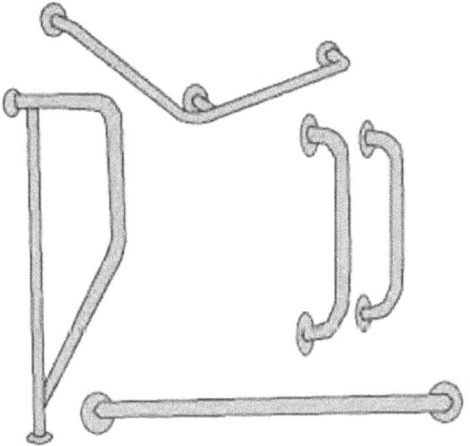

Points to Remember:
Movable grab bars on toilets minimize workplace congestion.
Ensure bars are securely fastened to wall before use.

Description:
Height adjustable shower gurney or lift bath cart with waterproof top.

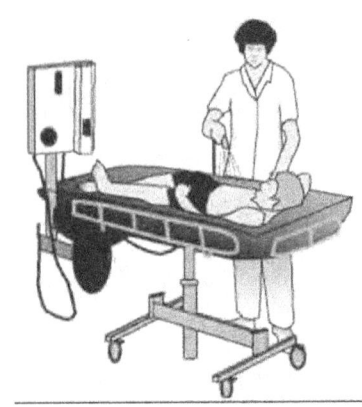

When to Use:
For bathing non-weight bearing residents who are unable to sit up. Transfer resident to cart with lift or lateral transfer boards or other friction-reducing devices.

Points to Remember:
The cart can be raised to eliminate bending and reaching to the caregiver. Foot and head supports are available for resident comfort. May not be suitable for bariatric residents. Look for carts that are power-driven to reduce force required to move and position device.

Description:
Built-in or fixed bath lifts.

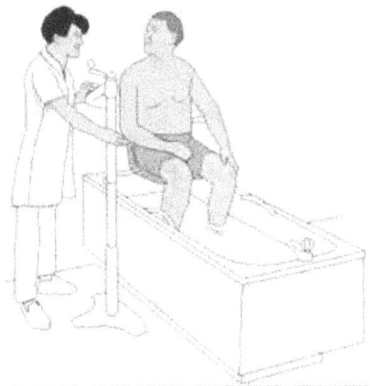

When to Use:
Bathing residents who are partially weight bearing, have good sitting balance, can use upper extremities (have upper body strength), are cooperative, and can follow instructions. Useful in small bathrooms where space is limited.

Points to Remember:
Ensure that seat raises so resident's feet clear tub, easily rotates, and lowers resident into water. May not be suitable for heavy residents. Always ensure lifting device is in good working order before use and rated for the resident weight. Choose device with lift mechanism that does not require excessive effort by caregiver when raising and lowering device.

A Identifying Problems and Implementing Solutions for Activities Other than Resident Lifting and Repositioning

Some reports indicate a significant number of work-related MSDs in nursing homes occur in activities other than resident lifting. (2, 3) Examples of some of the activities that the nursing home operator may want to review are:

- bending to make a bed or feed a resident;
- lifting food trays above shoulder level or below knee level;
- collecting waste;
- pushing heavy carts;
- bending to remove items from a deep cart;
- lifting and carrying when receiving and stocking supplies;
- bending and manually cranking an adjustable bed; and
- removing laundry from washing machines and dryers.

These tasks may not present problems in all circumstances. Employers should consider the duration, frequency, and magnitude of employee exposure to forceful exertions, repetitive activities, and awkward postures when determining if problems exist in these and other areas. In the vast majority of cases, job assessments can be accomplished by observing employees performing the task, by discussing with employees the activities and conditions that they associate with difficulties, and checking injury records. Observation provides general information about the workstation layout, tools, equipment, and general environmental conditions in the workplace. Discussing tasks with employees helps to ensure that a complete picture of the process is obtained. Employees who perform a given task are also often the best sources for identifying the cause of a problem, and developing the most practical and effective solutions. Once information is obtained and problems identified, suitable improvements can be implemented. Finally, there are a number of resources available to help determine if specific activities have the potential for causing injuries. For example, support is available from OSHA's consultation program, insurance companies, and state workers' compensation programs. The following are examples of possible solutions for activities other than resident lifting and repositioning.

Storage and Transfer of Food, Supplies, and Medications

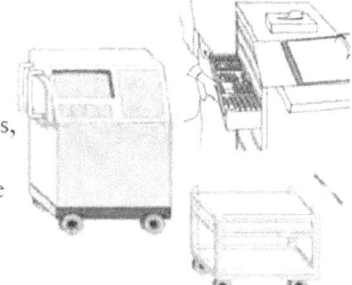

Description:
Use of carts.

When to Use:
When moving food trays, cleaning supplies, equipment, maintenance tools, and dispensing medications.

Points to Remember:
Speeds process for accessing and storing items. Placement of items on the cart should keep the most frequently used and heavy items within easy reach between hip and shoulder height. Carts should have full-bearing wheels of a material designed for the floor surface in your facility. Cart handles that are vertical, with some horizontal adjustability, will allow all employees to push at elbow height and shoulder width. Carts should have wheel locks. Handles that can swing out of the way may be useful for saving space or reducing reach. Heavy carts should have brakes. Balance loads and keep loads under cart weight restrictions. Ensure stack height does not block vision. Low profile medication carts with easy-open side drawers are recommended to accommodate hand height of shorter nurses.

Mobile Medical Equipment

Description:
Work methods and tools to transport equipment.

When to Use:
When transporting assistive devices and other equipment.

Points to Remember:
• Oxygen tanks: Use small cylinders with handles to reduce weight and allow for easier gripping. Secure oxygen tanks to transport device.
• Medication pumps: Use stands on wheels.
• Transporting equipment: Push equipment, rather than pull, when possible. Keep arms close to the body and push with whole body and not just arms. Remove unnecessary objects to minimize weight. Avoid obstacles that could cause abrupt stops. Place equipment on a rolling device if possible. Take defective equipment out of service. Perform routine maintenance on all equipment.
• Ensure that when moving and transporting residents, additional equipment such as oxygen tanks and IV/medication poles are attached to wheelchairs or gurneys or moved by another caregiver to avoid awkwardly pushing with one hand and holding freestanding equipment with the other hand.

Working with Liquids in Housekeeping

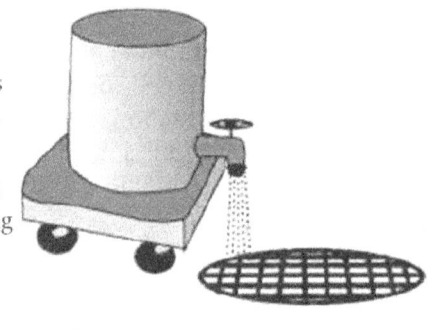

Description:
Filling and emptying liquids from containers.

When to Use:
In housekeeping areas when filling and emptying buckets with floor drain arrangements.

Points to Remember:
Reduces risk of spills, slips, speeds process, and reduces waste. The faucet and floor drain is used in housekeeping. Ensure that casters don't get stuck in floor grate. Use hose to fill bucket. Use buckets with casters to move mop bucket around. Ensure casters are maintained and roll easily.

Working with Liquids in Housekeeping

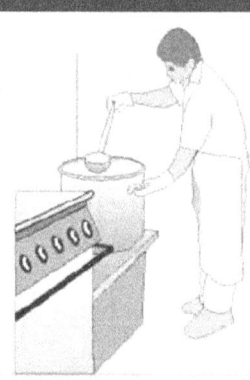

Description:
Filling and emptying liquids from containers.

When to Use:
In dietary when pouring soups or other liquid foods that are heavy.

Points to Remember:
Reduces risk of spills and burns, speeds process, and reduces waste.
Use an elevated faucet or hose to fill large pots. Avoid lifting heavy pots filled with liquids. Use ladle to empty liquids, soups, etc., from pots. Small sauce pans can also be used to dip liquids from pots. If the worker stands for more than 2 hours per day, shock-absorbing floors or insoles will minimize back and leg strain. With hot liquids, ensure a splash guard is included.

Hand Tools

Description:
Select and use properly designed tools.

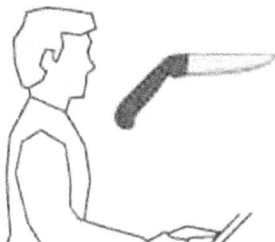

When to Use:
When selecting frequently used tools for the kitchen, housekeeping, laundry and maintenance areas.

Points to Remember:
Enhances tool safety, speeds process, and reduces waste. Handles should fit the grip size of the user. Use bent-handled tools to avoid bending wrists. Use appropriate tool weight. Select tools that have minimal vibration or vibration damping devices. Implement a regular maintenance program for tools to keep blades sharp and edges and handles intact. Always wear the appropriate personal protective equipment.

Linen Carts

Description:
Spring loaded carts that automatically bring linen within easy reach.

When to Use:
Moving or storing linen.

Points to Remember:
Speeds process for handling linen, and reduces wear on linen due to excessive pulling. Select a spring tension that is appropriate for the weight of the load. Carts should have wheel locks and height-appropriate handles that can swing out of the way. Heavy carts should have brakes.

Handling Bags

Description:
Equipment and practices for handling bags.

When to Use:
When handling laundry, trash, and other bags.

Points to Remember:
Reduces risk of items being dropped, and speeds process for removing and disposing of items. Receptacles that hold bags of laundry or trash should have side openings that keep the bags within easy reach and allow employees to slide the bag off the cart without lifting. Provide handles to decrease the strain of handling. Chutes and dumpsters should be positioned to minimize lifting. It is best to lower the dumpster or chute rather than lift materials to higher levels. Provide automatic opening or hardware to keep doors open to minimize twisting and awkward handling.

Reaching into Sink

Description:
Tools used to modify a deep sink for cleaning small objects.

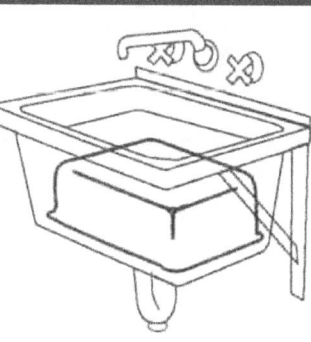

When to Use:
Cleaning small objects in a deep sink.

Points to Remember:
Place an object such as a plastic basin in the bottom of the sink to raise the work surface. An alternative is to use a smaller porous container to hold small objects for soaking, transfer to an adjacent countertop for aggressive cleaning, and then transfer back to the sink for final rinsing. Store inserts and containers in a convenient location to encourage consistent use. This technique is not suitable in kitchens/food preparation.

Loading or Unloading Laundry

Description:
Front-loading washers and dryers.

When to Use:
When loading or unloading laundry from washers, dryers and other laundry equipment.

Points to Remember:
Speeds process for retrieving and placing items, and minimizes wear-and-tear on linen. Washers with tumbling cycles separate clothes, making removal easier. For deep tubs, a rake with long or extendable handle can be used to pull linen closer to the door opening. Raise machines so that opening is between hip and elbow height of employees. If using top loading washers, work practices that reduce risk include handling small loads of laundry, handling only a few items at a time, and bracing your body against the front of the machine when lifting. If items are knotted in the machine, brace with one hand while using the other to gently pull the items free. Ensure that items go into a cart rather than picking up baskets of soiled linen or wet laundry.

Cleaning Rooms (Electrical)

Description:
Work methods and tools to vacuum and buff floors.

When to Use:
Vacuuming and buffing floors.

Points to Remember:
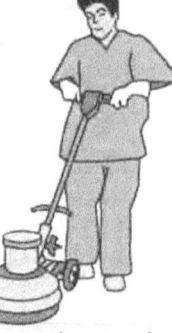
• Both vacuum cleaners and buffers should have lightweight construction, adjustable handles, triggers (buffer) long enough to accommodate at least the index and middle fingers, and easy to reach controls. Technique is important for both devices, including use of appropriate grips, avoiding tight grips, and for vacuuming, by alternating grip. The use of telescoping and extension handles, hoses, and tools can reduce reaching for low areas, high areas, and far away areas. Maintain and service the equipment and change vacuum bags when 1/2 to 3/4 full.
• Vacuums and other powered devices are preferred over manual equipment for moderate-to-long duration use. Heavy canisters or other large, heavy equipment should have brakes.

Cleaning Rooms (Wet Method)

Description:
Work methods and tools to clean resident rooms with water and chemical products.

When to Use:
When cleaning with water and chemical products and using spray bottles.

Points to Remember:
• Cleaning implement: use alternate leading hand, avoid tight static grip and use padded non-slip handles.
• Spray bottles: Use trigger handles long enough for the index and middle fingers. Avoid using the ring and little fingers.
• For all cleaning: Use chemical cleaners and abrasive sponges to minimize scrubbing force. Use kneepads when kneeling. Avoid bending and twisting. Use extension handles, step stools, or ladders for overhead needs. Use carts to transport supplies or carry only small quantities and weights of supplies. Ventilation of rooms may be necessary when chemicals are used.
• Avoid lifting heavy buckets, e.g., lifting a large, full bucket from a sink. Use a hose or similar device to fill buckets with water. Use wheels on buckets that roll easily and have functional brakes. Ensure that casters are maintained. Use rubber-soled shoes in wet areas to prevent slipping.
• Cleaning wheelchairs: Cleaning workstation should be at appropriate height.

Training

Training is critical for employers and employees to safely use the suggestions identified in these guidelines. Of course, training should be provided in a manner and language that all employees can understand. The following describes areas of training for nursing home employees, their supervisors, and program managers who are responsible for planning and managing the nursing home's ergonomics efforts. OSHA recommends refresher training be provided as needed to reinforce initial training and to address new developments in the workplace.

Nursing Assistants and Other Workers at Risk of Injury

Employees should be trained before they lift or reposition residents, or perform other work that may involve risk of injury. Ergonomics training can be included with other safety and health training, or incorporated into general instructions provided to employees. Training is usually most effective when it includes case studies or demonstrations based on the nursing home's polices, and allows enough time to answer any questions that may arise. Training should ensure that these workers understand:

- policies and procedures that should be followed to avoid injury, including proper work practices and use of equipment;
- how to recognize MSDs and their early indications;
- the advantages of addressing early indications of MSDs before serious injury has developed; and
- the nursing home's procedures for reporting work-related injuries and illnesses as required by OSHA's injury and illness recording and reporting regulation (29 CFR 1904).

Training for Charge Nurses and Supervisors

Charge nurses and supervisors should reinforce the safety program of the facility, oversee reporting guidelines, and help ensure the implementation of resident and task specific ergonomics recommendations, e.g., using a mechanical lift. Because charge nurses and supervisors are likely to receive reports of injuries, and are usually responsible for implementing the nursing home's work practices, they may need more detailed training than nursing assistants on:

- methods for ensuring use of proper work practices;
- how to respond to injury reports; and
- how to help other workers implement solutions.

Training for Designated Program Managers

Staff members who are responsible for planning and managing ergonomics efforts need training so they can identify ergonomics concerns and select appropriate solutions. These staff members should receive information and training that will allow them to:

- identify potential problems related to physical activities in the workplace through observation, use of checklists, injury data analysis, or other analytical tools;
- address problems by selecting proper equipment and work practices;
- help other workers implement solutions; and
- evaluate the effectiveness of ergonomics efforts.

SECTION VI
Additional Sources of Information

The following sources may be useful to those seeking further information about ergonomics and the prevention of work-related MSDs in nursing homes.

A Back Injury Prevention Guide for Health Care Providers, Cal/OSHA Consultation Programs, (800) 963-9424, www.dir.ca.gov/dosh/dosh_publications/backinj.pdf This guide discusses the scope of the back injury problem in health care, how to analyze the workplace, how to identify and implement improvements, and how to evaluate results. It includes checklists that can assist in analyzing the work environment.

Patient Care Ergonomics Resource Guide: Safe Patient Handling and Movement, Patient Safety Center of Inquiry, Veterans Health Administration and Department of Defense, (813) 558-3902, www.patientsafetycenter.com This document describes a comprehensive program developed to prevent MSDs related to resident lifting and repositioning. It includes assessment criteria and flowcharts for selecting equipment and techniques for safe lifting and repositioning based on resident characteristics.

Resident Assessment Instrument, U.S. Department of Health and Human Services - Centers for Medicareand Medicaid Services (CMS), www.cms.hhs.gov/medicaid/mds20/ This document is used by many nursing homes to evaluate resident needs and capabilities.

Elements of Ergonomics Programs, U.S. Department of Health and Human Services - National Institute for Occupational Safety and Health, (800) 356-4674, www.cdc.gov/niosh/ephome2.html The basic elements of a workplace program aimed at preventing work-related musculoskeletal disorders are described in this document. It includes a "toolbox," which is a collection of techniques, methods, reference materials, and sources for other information that can help in program development.

In addition, OSHAC's Training Institute in Arlington Heights, Illinois, offers courses on various safety and health topics, including ergonomics. Courses are also offered through Training Institute Education Centers located throughout the country. For a schedule of courses, contact the OSHA Training Institute, 2020 South Arlington Heights Road, Arlington Heights, Illinois, 60005, (847) 297-4810, or visit OSHA's training resources webpage at www.osha.gov. Choose "Training" from the blue column on the right, under Compliance Assistance.

Additional Sources of Information

There are many states and territories that operate their own occupational safety and health programs under a plan approved by OSHA (23 cover both private sector, state and local government employees, and three only cover public employees). See the map on www.osha.gov for information on how to contact a state plan directly for information about specific state nursing home initiatives and compliance assistance, or state standards that may apply to nursing homes.

A free consultation service is available to provide occupational safety and health assistance to businesses. OSHA Consultation is funded primarily by federal OSHA but delivered by the 50 state governments, the District of Columbia, Guam, Puerto Rico, and the Virgin Islands. The states offer the expertise of highly qualified occupational safety and health professionals to employers who request help to establish and maintain a safe and healthful workplace. Developed for small and medium-sized employers in hazardous industries or with hazardous operations, the service is provided at no cost to the employer and is confidential. Information on OSHA consultation can be found at www.osha.gov. Choose "Consultation" from the blue column at the right under Compliance Assistance, or request the booklet *Consultation Services for the Employer* (OSHA 3047) from OSHA's Publications Office at (202) 693-1888.

More information on ergonomics and other safety and health issues is available on OSHA's website at www.osha.gov. See the index at the top of the home page. For any additional information regarding Guidelines for Nursing Homes, please contact the OSHA's Directorate of Standards and Guidance at 202-693-1950.

References

(1) Documents submitted to OSHA by Wyandot County Nursing Home. (Ex. 3-12)

(2) Garg, A. 1999. Long-Term Effectiveness of "Zero-Lift Program" in Seven Nursing Homes and One Hospital. U.S. Department of Health and Human Services, Centers for Disease Control and Prevention, National Institute for Occupational Safety and Health (NIOSH), Cincinnati, OH. August. Contract No. U60/CCU512089-02. (Ex. 3-3)

(3) Fragala, G., PhD, PE, CSP. 1996. Ergonomics: How to Contain On-the-Job Injuries in Health Care. Joint Commission on Accreditation of Healthcare Organizations.

(4) Occupational Safety and Health Administration, Region II. Summer, 2002. New York OSHA E-Newsletter, Vol. 1, Issue 2.

(5) National Institute for Occupational Safety and Health (NIOSH). 1997. Musculoskeletal Disorders and Workplace Factors - A Critical Review of Epidemiologic Evidence for Work-Related Musculoskeletal Disorders of the Neck, Upper Extremity, and Low Back. (Ex. 3-4)

(6) National Research Council and Institute of Medicine. 2001. Musculoskeletal Disorders and the Workplace - Low Back and Upper Extremities. National Academy of Sciences. Washington, DC: National Academy Press. (Ex. 3-6)

(7) Taylor and Francis. 1988. Cumulative Trauma Disorders: A Manual for MSDs of the Upper Limb. Putz-Anderson, V., ed.

(8) Documents submitted to OSHA by Citizens Memorial. (Ex. 3-25)

(9) U.S. General Accounting Office. 1997. Worker Protection - Private Sector Ergonomics Programs Yield Positive Results. August. GAO/HEHS-97-163. (Ex. 3-92)

(10) American Health Care Association, American Association of Homes and Services for the Aging, National Center for Assisted Living. 2002. Comments submitted to OSHA. (Ex. 4-15)

Appendix - A Nursing Home Case Study

Introduction

Wyandot County Nursing Home used a process that reflects many of the recommendations in these guidelines to address safety and health concerns and phase-in its current program that entails no manual lifting of residents. First and foremost, Wyandot's administrator provided strong commitment and support in addressing the home's problems. He also involved Wyandot's workers in every phase of the effort. He talked to his employees, learned about stressful parts of their jobs, and then found solutions. He and his employees identified existing and potential sources of injury at the home and worked to implement solutions. He trained employees each time the nursing home introduced new equipment. He continually checked new equipment, and he continues to evaluate the overall effectiveness of his safety and health efforts. Wyandot is located in Upper Sandusky, Ohio. It is a 100-bed, county-run facility that has served Wyandot County in its present building for the past 28 years. It is divided into two sections to serve residents with different levels of need. The A- wing, with 32 rooms, serves residents who are mostly ambulatory and require only a minimum of help with daily living.

This case study was developed from information provided by Wyandot County Nursing Home. OSHA visited the nursing home to discuss the ergonomics program with the nursing home administrator, observe ergonomics corrective actions, and talk to employees, residents, and family members about their experiences.

In the B- and C- wings, with 32 double rooms and four private ones, residents receive care that ranges from extensive to total. Wyandot has 90 employees, 45 of whom are nursing assistants. This makes for a nursing staff ratio of 2.4 hours for each resident per day.

Identifying Problems

Before Wyandot implemented its ergonomics program, the home was experiencing problems that were a growing concern to both the county and Wyandot's administrator. According to Wyandot, workers' compensation costs averaged almost $140,000 per year from 1995-1997. The turnover rate among nursing assistants averaged over 55 percent during that same time period. This meant that of the 45 nursing assistants working at Wyandot, on average 25 new ones had to be hired each year.

Wyandot's administrator began to look for more effective ways to address injuries among workers and the high turnover rate. A back injury suffered by a worker that cost Wyandot $240,000 in workers' compensation expenses provided significant motivation to find a strategy that would work. As Wyandot's administrator investigated that injury, he also examined other sources of potential injury within the home. In doing so, he learned that resident transfer and repositioning tasks presented high risks for injuries.

He called on the Ohio Bureau of Workers' Compensation (OBWC) for help because he thought Wyandot was following best practices and people were still being injured. An OBWC ergonomist visited the home and told him that he had unrealistic expectations about his nursing staff's ability to manually lift and reposition residents.

Involving Employees

Wyandot's administrator thought that he could better use his existing staff. After hearing about a "no lift" policy and seeing an impressive demonstration of mechanical lifts at an industry conference, he began to consider setting up a program at Wyandot. He became convinced that such a program would keep employees safer and help slow the turnover rate while ensuring safety and high quality care for residents.

He decided that the best approach was to involve employees at every level in reducing injuries and slowing the turnover rate. More than 30 workers volunteered to examine the tasks of moving and repositioning residents.

Wyandot employees concluded that better body mechanics — the traditional method of lifting and transferring residents at most nursing homes — was not the answer. In fact, he and his staff determined that there was no safe way to lift a resident other than with mechanical lifts. To determine what equipment would work best, Wyandot tried out various pieces of equipment, evaluated each lift, and then decided what would be most appropriate for Wyandot's needs.

Implementing Solutions

With recommendations from employees, Wyandot's administrator bought several portable mechanical lifts for the B- and C-wings. These involved portable sit-to-stand lifts, walk/ambulating lifts, and total lifts. Nurses and assistants could move each of these from room to room as they worked with individual residents. However, many of the staff remained unconvinced of the value of using equipment. In fact, initially only the workers who had actually evaluated the lifts were using them.

According to Wyandot's administrator, it was very difficult getting workers to overcome their insistence on doing things the old way. Because many workers said it took too long to use the mechanical lifts, one of the co-charge nurses decided to do a time study. She wanted to test how long it took to lift a resident manually compared to using a mechanical lift. The mechanical lift took about 5 minutes. Meanwhile, to perform the manual lift, a nursing assistant first had to find someone to help. This took 15 minutes. Thus, the time study showed that using the equipment actually saved time.

One worker, who admitted that she did not initially use the sit-tostand lift because it was a "hassle," reconsidered her opinion after an outbreak of the flu reduced the number of staff members available for assistance. In her words, "I was forced to use the lift. Awesome. It was just great. I was so sorry my fellow employees had to suffer with the flu bug to get me to use this contraption."

Wyandot's administrator also wanted to replace the old hand-crank beds at Wyandot with electric beds. To do this, he also needed to find beds that would be used in the "low-bed" system in place for many residents. There were not many options available, so he took his ideas and engineering background to a bed company and inquired about having beds designed to fit Wyandot's needs. The bed manufacturer designed the new beds to lift from the floor to a height of about 30 inches in 20 seconds. In addition, these fast beds were designed so that residents would be less likely to slide to the foot of the bed as they were raised to a sitting position. As a result, residents would not need to be repositioned. Also, the beds could be used with a gait-belt for ambulatory residents to assist them from a sitting to a standing position.

About three years after Wyandot began its ergonomics effort, the nursing home received a grant from the OBWC Division of Safety and Hygiene through an ergonomic emphasis program to deal with cumulative trauma disorders. The grant enabled Wyandot's administrator to purchase 58 fast electric beds, a turning point for staff acceptance. When the first ceiling lifts were installed seven months later, employees were ready to use them.

One nursing assistant, who has been with Wyandot for 19 years, explained why she liked the new beds so much. "We can quickly bring the bed up to our work height with a push of a button and we can reposition a resident . . . with ease without stooping or struggling."

The final phase of Wyandot's program began with the introduction of the ceiling lifts. Wyandot's administrator evaluated several ceiling lift systems. Wyandot chose a system with a motorized lift and a ceiling mounted track. Tracks were retrofitted into the rooms at a cost of about $12,000 for two double rooms and one bathroom. The first double room had a track that extended into the bathroom. However, newer systems used a transfer between the room and bathroom, which simplified the system and reduced costs.

Providing Training

As Wyandot purchased and installed new equipment, workers received training on how to use it, and guidelines for equipment use were put into place. An LPN in-service director did the training. New employees learned how to use the devices and knew where to go for further instruction or help. Eventually, most of the nursing assistants adapted to the mechanical lifts and refused to use any other lifting techniques.

Providing Management Support

Wyandot's administrator took a personal interest in ergonomic issues. To address high injury and turnover rates at Wyandot, he remained committed to identifying and solving problems. For example, on one occasion the staff said that the lifts were not easy to roll on the floors in the B- and C- wings. To solve the problem, he experimented with different wheels that would roll more easily and turn in tight places with less effort. Finally, he worked with a manufacturer to find and buy better casters to suit the home's flooring.

Evaluating Efforts

To start with, Wyandot's administrator spent $150,000 to buy equipment. He later set aside another $130,000 to continue his efforts, for a total of $280,000. Wyandot has saved $55,000 annually in payroll costs, according to

Appendix

Wyandot's administrator, because of reduced overtime and absenteeism. The home estimates savings of more than $125,000 in turnover costs. Meanwhile, workers' compensation costs also have fallen drastically. For example, Wyandot reports that, after the program was implemented workers' compensation costs declined from an average of $140,000 per year to less than $4,000 per year.

From the time workers began to use the sit-to-stand lifts, which were among the first to be introduced at Wyandot, the incidence of back injuries stopped. Once the fast beds were introduced only six new hires were needed in the following year.

Worker satisfaction has increased greatly. One nursing assistant, who has spent most of her career working in nursing homes, confessed to being sore and unhappy at Wyandot before the lifts were introduced. After the innovations at the nursing home, she reported that she is no longer hurting. She concluded that "I think my career is right here in the Wyandot County Nursing Home till my time is due to retire comfortable. And you know if my time comes to be in a nursing home I do hope I get one like ours."

Mechanical lifts have also helped return a sense of dignity to Wyandot's residents. As one nursing assistant put it, through the use of the mechanical lifts, the residents are able to wear normal clothing again, which "improves their self-esteem and keeps them warmer."

The wife of one totally dependent resident who has been at Wyandot for eight years reports that because of her husband's size, he cannot help the nurses and nursing assistants in moving him from place to place. Before the overhead electric lifts and electric beds were installed in his room, it took three and sometimes four nursing assistants to move him from the bed to his cart or to the toilet. He had numerous bruises from falling and dreaded being moved. With the lifts in place, the resident's wife reports that the staff "can easily move him about to his chair and to the toilet. He cannot sit without help but the sling gives him comfortable support and makes it possible to have some dignity."